The Natural Solution To Diabetes & Prediabetes

How To Manage Low & High Blood Sugar, Diet For Weight Loss & Nutrition, And Handle The Eating, Cooking & Living Connection

By Jerry Reaves

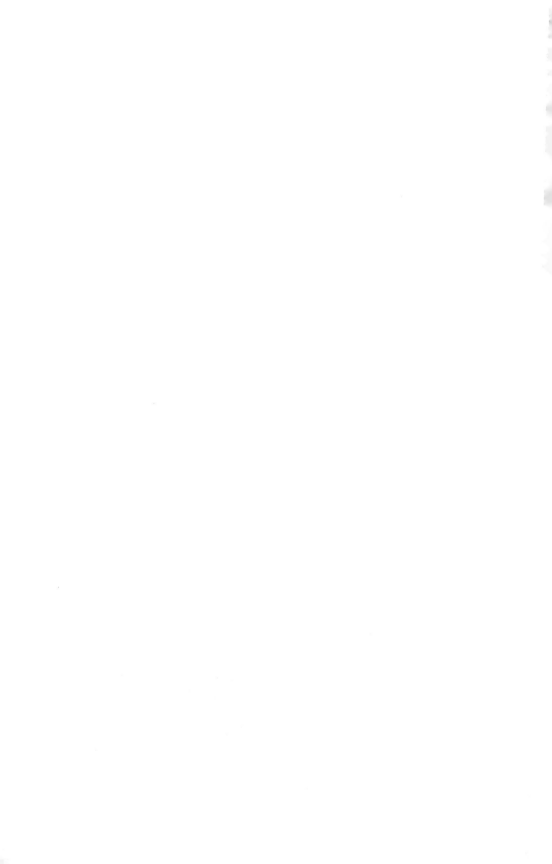

The Natural Solution To Diabetes and Prediabetes: How To Manage Low & High Blood Sugar, Diet For Weight Loss & Nutrition, and Handle The Eating, Cooking & Living Connection

By Jerry Reaves

Legal Stuff

Table of Contents

Introduction

5 years ago, I was working for one of the biggest banks in America as a loan consultant when I had this terrible news from my health care provider. It was after my colleagues and I underwent the annual physical examination when a doctor diagnosed me of having a metabolic syndrome. He deemed that I was a prediabetic.

At that point, I was all ears. Like many of us, I had no idea what this doctor is saying and it just made sense to me when the word diabetes was observed. Nevertheless, I'll admit that even after he had bombarded me with terms that are alien to me like hyperglycemia, glucose, blood plasma, insulin resistance, pancreatic beta cells and whatnot, the fact that I have developed a disease didn't sink in to me like a shot.

What happened was that I was trying to catch up with the words the health care provider is throwing at me. He mentioned drugs that I now need to take for medication. I was told that I now have to be familiar with insulin, where can I get it, how should it be properly injected. He also recommended some more people who are specialists in blood sugar management that I needed to see.

I'm fortunate that there is a bit of a stubbornness in me that tries to determine the answer to every question myself. I knew that the most important words that fell from my healthcare providers was when he told me that I needed to learn everything there is to know about diabetes. If I am to succeed in living the happy life I'm enjoying now even with this condition at the back of my head, I needed to become an expert at it.

Now here's the clincher, "Do you truly think that your healthcare provider wants you to become an expert at your newfound ordeal even on topics like alternative medicine?"

For me, I felt that the answer to that question is "NO". The realization came of course when I was back at home and by myself.

It came to me that no matter how genuinely helpful a healthcare provider's medication may be, we shouldn't turn away from the fact that they are running a business. Hold that idea and think whether that form of business can benefit from giving out medicines derived from plants. Likewise, will it serve their business' interest by handing out a list of foods that naturally fights the spell cast by diabetes? Having said that, I've learned that it isn't the health care system's fault for focusing on profit generating cures rather than more cost-effective lifestyle changes and natural alternative medicine even though they can work just as fine. They have no choice because that's how every other business is programmed – to generate profit.

This is when I made the commitment to discover supplements, natural diets, and every lifehacks I can find to integrate into my lifestyle to better combat this disease. This book contains the cherry-picked information that has helped me ever since learning about them through many hours of offline and online research.

If you also thought that it was weird that someone is telling you to become an expert at something yet dictates all the (expensive) solutions you could use, this book offers an entirely new method that you may prefer to take.

Chapter 1: What Is Diabetes?

Insulin is a type of hormone that our body naturally produce to allow our body cells to consume sugar. Diabetes occurs when a condition exists wherein either not enough insulin is being produced or it no longer is effective at doing its job because the body has built up a resistance to it.

In most cases, diabetes is genetically linked. This implies that there is no one to blame. If what you have is type 1 diabetes, you've had it since you were very young because it was passed on to you through the genes of your parents. When a person is diagnosed of having this, the initial medication responses he or she will get are from healthcare workers, whom will tell you that in order to survive; you'll have to start relying on external insulin source.

Diabetes type 2 is the instance where the body is producing insulin, but the body is resisting the natural effects it should have in the bodily functions. In most cases, this is coupled with the relatively insufficient secretion of the hormone as well. This type of diabetes is the most widespread.

What Causes It?

Researches are quick to point out that adults who are affected with this metabolic abnormality may have developed the conditions because of the following:

- An illness
- An accident
- Diet
- Lifestyle

Whatever diabetes type a person may have, the root of the problem always is that the body's cells aren't receiving enough insulin. Although insufficient insulin production isn't a threat condition on its own, its effects in the body are catastrophic. Without it, the cells in our body doesn't receive the glucose that they need for maintenance and repairs.

Glucose is a form of simple sugar that by far is the most preferred fuel of our body cells. Without it, the body would soon begin to deteriorate. This explains the common symptoms of diabetes such as wounds not healing, amputation of limbs, and even blindness (many do not recognize that diabetes is the leading cause of blindness). So what does insulin have to do with our body not consuming glucose? Everything. It's the catastrophic effect I was telling you about. Insulin is the catalyst between the absorption of glucose into our body cells. With the catalyst removed from the picture, our body doesn't get the supply that it needs in order to maintain itself from the day-to-day beating.

What Are Its Effects?

Here's another bad news, the body doesn't stop the seething of glucose. Every time we time we eat, an amount of glucose is formed and introduced into our blood stream. It's a part of digestion that we have no workaround. There is no off button for this because our body should be able to constantly feed off this supply. For people who have diabetes, where do you think does your glucose go?

It stays where it is initially dumped – in our blood. Therefore, if left unattended, the blood could easily be oversaturated with sugar where it would wreak havoc such as strokes, heart attacks, blindness, damage to kidneys and limbs.

Despite the always-on database of health information on the internet, diabetes still affects 8% of the world's population. Moreover, year over year, that statistic continues to worsen. Throughout my ordeal with diabetes, I have learned that the same technological advancements we are enjoying is both the key solution and the major cause of the problem. Our lifestyle of being entertained while on the couch, automated gadgetries simplifying our chores and lack of physical activities are taking its toll on our body's systems, which are designed for an entirely different style of living. I desire to help anyone who reads this book to get back into that latter way of living, which will assist in your fight with diabetes the natural way.

Chapter 2: The Diabetic Diet – Your Food Cheat Sheet That Fights Diabetes

Learn About the Fullness Factor (Glycemic Index)

There is more to the dichotomy of carbohydrates than meets the eye. In fact, it's not as basic as knowing simply how to distinguish between these two main categories of carbohydrates – simple and complex. Simple carbohydrates are normally found in maple syrup, honey and sugar. Complex carbohydrates include fruits, vegetables, legumes, and whole grain foods. We were brought up knowing that we should reduce simple sugars from our diet and get more from the complex carbohydrates platter. Still, it's far more complicated than that.

How Does Simple Becomes Complex?

It is indeed a paradox how something simple can actually be complex. But when you are diagnosed with diabetes, you most likely turn into a geek as you nervously fidget across the keyboards to explore and search about the advanced treatments, alternative routes, as well as the most up-to-date and detailed information regarding your health condition. It's fascinating how a pre-diabetic diagnosis can change your life and rattle your existence to the point of paranoia. I am not exaggerating by the way.

Let's see how simple dichotomy is not really a clear-cut channel.

Aside from identifying these two classes of carbohydrate, we should also recognize how fast a rate and how high a certain carbohydrate can metabolize into sugar enough to impact glucose levels at certain points – that is coined as glycemic index (GI) levels. Blood sugar, which is delivered through the bloodstream into varied organs of the body that is stored as energy, is in part derived from carbohydrates. On average, a food with low glycemic index (GI) usually raises the blood sugar at a tolerable level while food classified under high glycemic index (GI) can potentially increase blood sugar level to extreme points.

The irony is that there are some complex carbohydrates that surprisingly belong to the high GI category such as potatoes that is recognized as a healthy carbohydrate. This becomes the superficial role of mapping out a diet plan. Rather than sticking with the snappy identification of complex and simple carbohydrates, which turns out to be pretty unreliable – the GI values bears more weight in the selection process of what certain foods can tick off the sugar levels and what does not. The GI values then are vital information in choosing the proper food that can put glucose levels under control.

What is the Glycemic Index (GI)?

The Glycemic Index (GI) is referred to as numerical scale, which is used to rank and determined certain food that can affect blood sugar levels. Awareness of the GI levels of certain food groups can help you moderate glucose levels. Food with high GI levels can optimize the glucose levels to a hazardous extent while food groups under the low GI levels are below normal or safe glucose levels. Combining certain GI levels of food categories can level off the sugar levels at a certain extent. Many people use the GI classification for weight loss, controlling diabetes, reducing cholesterol levels, and preventing heart diseases; to name a few.

Carbohydrate – Rich Food Groups:

Sugars – These are classified into those found in dairy products and fruits as well as he processed sugars and sweeteners available in the market.

Fiber – This does not directly tweak the blood sugar levels because, and peas, starchy vegetables (yams, squash, and potatoes), and grains (rice, barley, and wheat).

These above carbohydrate – rich food categories are usually what we hunger for when we are stressed out or sustaining the "blues" – which is precisely why these are labelled as "comfort foods". These are likewise regarded as staple food in most countries.

Carbohydrates actually have that vital effect on glucose levels that starts from digestion wherein they are broken up and turned into glucose, which can readily ride into our blood stream and onto varied organ systems. Proteins and fats are relatively not broken down into glucose by the same process so they typically have less effect on glucose levels than carbohydrates.

Glucose in the bloodstream can set off insulin production that is a hormone that aids blood sugar to penetrate the cells wherein it can be immediately used for energy. Once the body's need for energy boosts have been satisfied, the remaining glucose in our blood stream is stored in the liver and muscles intended for later use. Now, if the muscles and liver are filled with glucose and yet there is still spare glucose in the bloodstream, then the insulin acts by storing this excess glucose as fat. Now we know how the blood sugar level is directly related to obesity. Cutting down on sugar and carbs literally and figuratively is important in maintaining that sexy hourglass figure while reducing risks for cardiovascular diseases.

Insulin production is definitely a good factor because it helps the glucose get into the cells to initiate energy production. But, too much insulin released in our body over extended period of time can cause more health trouble. Research data indicates that increased levels of insulin can potentially result in the following:

- Obesity
- Hypertension
- Insulin Resistance
- Risk of Aggravating or Developing Type 2 Diabetes
- Low triglyceride
- Levels Low HDL (Good) Cholesterol
- High LDL (Bad) Cholesterol
- Increased Appetite Levels

The danger seethes in with the combination of these factors, which is coined as the metabolic syndrome. The existence of all these factors can escalate a person's risk level for a wide range of cardiovascular diseases, cancer, and diabetes. A single high load of GI meal may not instigate significant health issues but habits and prolonged ingestion of high GI load meals can boost the insulin levels to a dangerous range. When the insulin levels remain very high, the endocrine system can go ballistic as it struggles to adapt to the amplified insulin levels along with the erratic hormonal shifts that can leave you thirsty and fatigued, which eventually sets you off on a collision course with type 2 diabetes and heart diseases.

We are all into the candy rush and chocolate – dubbed as "food of the gods". They say it's an aphrodisiac or a cure for a massive heartbreak. Whichever way, cravings for too many sweets can either lead you to insulin surges, a toothache, or your hormones gone berserk. Do you feel some hormonal shook-up or lethargy after eating a pack of your favourite candy or a box of donuts?

You might feel an impacting jolt that causes hyperactivity followed by increased fatigue. This occurs when there is too much insulin in the blood stream that triggers hypoglycaemia or low blood sugar, which leads to you having low energy.

On the other hand, consuming a low GI load meal can stabilize both glucose and insulin levels at a non-alarming rate. Basically, low GI load meals have a radically slower digestion and absorption rate than its counterpart; which means the nutrients are released progressively that keeps the blood sugar and insulin levels at bay.

When you do not have an idea that food choices are crucial to your energy levels, you tend to consume the same meals on a day-to-day grind that loads up your system with too much glucose to the point of exhaustion. Your system can crash with this kind of lifestyle. I, for one, have cravings for sweets and I used to believe that this could give me the energy boost that I need for my everyday tasks. I pop a candy when I felt sleepy or much on chocolate bars when I feel depressed or anxious. And I get anxious radically most of the time.

So you could only imagine how many of these delectable and tempting sweets I consume everyday then. True enough, it gives me that incredible shake to ward off my laziness and get back to crunch time but it eventually hits me back by surprise and leaves me tired and craving for more. Makes me wonder sometimes if this is part of a cruel advertising tempo or just me and my crazy hormones deluding me to an oh-so-sweet addiction?

Well, it's all about you and your food choice. You are what you eat right? Eating the low GI mode is definitely the surefire route to beating diabetic. Robert Crahyon, author of the Paleolithic Diet explains that there are two carbohydrate groups:

- Neo Carbs – these are the so-called agricultural carbohydrates that are primarily composed of flour, legumes, and grains, which have relatively high GI levels.

- Paleo Carbs – this type of carbohydrates is said to be the primary life sustenance of early people, which are generally found to have a low GI.

Most of the varieties found in the World's Healthiest Foods consist mainly of paleo carbs. The trick to getting the best of both worlds is in moderation. Striking the perfect balance between eating low GI and high GI meals can be dome. Our grocery carts could definitely tell how much of these foods we tend to prepare and eat each meal. This would be very difficult and tasking to plan especially because most of these ingredients are a steady mux of the low GI level food and that of the high GI varieties.

It's definitely a relief to know that we can still enjoy meals with higher GI levels as long as we balance it off with low GI foods. For instance, I love banana (which presumably coined to be a complete food but is now categorically placed at the high GI level plate). You can prepare it with your favorite oatmeal and moderate sugar levels with a toss of some seeds or nuts (which has incredibly low GI levels) and a generous sprinkle of cinnamon, which is said to improve the ability of the cells to absorb glucose.

How Do You Simplify and Estimate the Glycemic Index (GI) Of Food?

The glycemic Index (GI) levels of food can somewhat be trivial especially for a non-dietitian like me who rarely cooks and just eat what's in the fridge, heat it up, and presto! – A meal. And if all else fails, I prefer food delivery – it's quick, simple, and convenient. How do we simplify health when we are dealing with broad quantity levels of glucose and biochemical processes that happen with digestion? I feel like I'm having the dizzy spells just thinking of how you can effectively quantify whether a certain food group has low or high GI levels. Here are no-brainer tips to estimate GI levels with meals:

Food color matters. Food that are white usually have high glycemic index (GI) levels. This would include a variety of processed foods that are made with the use of white sugar or white flour.

Focus On Eating Fiber-Rich Foods. You will never go wrong with eating foods that are high in fiber. It is best to go for the unprocessed foods that has high quantity levels of fiber because these take much longer to digest which also lead to slower surge of blood glucose and insulin levels. This then makes you feel full much longer that prevents binge eating. Most of the World's Healthiest Foods are relatively high in fiber such as legumes, vegetables, nuts, whole grains, and citrus fruits, which are advisable to be eaten with the pulp and not as a smoothie or juice.

Go For A Protein-Rich Diet. Opt for organic substances with less fat, which contain a generous portion of omega-3 fatty and not the saturated fats that can precipitate certain life-threatening diseases such as cancer and cardiovascular conditions. Legumes; for instance, are rich in both fiber and protein that gives you double the buffer you need health wise. Other protein-rich foods include fish, nuts, seeds and lean meats.

Turn To The Healthy Fat – fats would often raise eyebrows. But not all fat variants are deemed unhealthy and could raise caloric levels, make you obese and shook up your entire body system with risk factors for heart conditions and other lifestyle diseases. Turning to the healthy fat or the omega-3 fats and monounsaturated fats in certain food options will boost your health. The healthy fat can be found in nuts, flaxseed oils, fish and olive oil.

An Individual's Glycemic Response Will Depend On Not Just One Food Variety But All The Rest Of Foods Consumed Alongside It. Be Sure To Eat a "Complex" Meal. Complex meals help balance your consumption especially if you thrive on variety – which is a good thing. This also keeps your blood glucose levels at a steady rate. Basically, a complex meal would have a myriad of complex carbohydrates such as fruits, vegetables, and whole grains, as well as a healthy dose of good fats, protein and fiber.

Now, that doesn't sound too complicated right? These are doable tips that you can work on every meal whether you decide to eat out or test your culinary prowess. I realized too (especially now that I have this pre-diabetic condition) that I should learn how to cook as this is one of the most defined ways to take control of my health as well as of those around me. That should pretty much go on top of my to-do-list for the year and probably another book on that.

Superfoods for Diabetes

With the basics in mind and the glycemic index (GI) levels scrutinized, we can now map out the diet plan that will work on diabetes that mesh well with our lifestyle, budget, health, condition, and taste preference. Every meal plan should be customized to get individual dietary needs and mist has apt proportions. Superfoods are naturally rich in vitamins A, C, and E, magnesium, calcium, fiber, and potassium.

Here are the top 10 Superfoods for Diabetes:

Dark Green Leafy Vegetables – you can never have too much vegetables especially with this kind. Dark leafy veggies have very low levels of carbohydrates and calories. You can never go wrong with this in your menu. You can choose among the kale, spinach and collards to name a few.

Beans – these are also considered as starchy vegetables. You can pick among the black, navy, kidney, or pinto beans – whichever you prefer. All beans are considered nutritious, as these are very rich in fiber content. More so, this is considered to be a rich source of potassium and magnesium. A half cup of noodles is enough to provide you about ½ of daily dietary requirement. This makes you feel full longer and prevents glucose levels from spiking, especially after meals.

Sweet Potatoes – this is a great alternative to the regular potatoes because it has a lower GI level. This is also packed with health benefits from fiber to vitamin A.

Citrus Fruits – these are best consumed with the whole produce – together with the pulp. Juice takes out a good deal of the fiber in the process and even some of the vital nutrients with it; leaving behind the sugar and calories. It is recommended to have 3-4 servings each day. You can take a dice, slice of oranges, limes, grapefruit, and lemons, and get your daily-recommended dose of vitamin C, fiber, and antioxidants.

Tomatoes – No matter how you prep your tomatoes (raw, pureed, or in sauce form), you will have the same dose of essential nutrients such as iron, vitamin C, and vitamin E.

Berries – this is definitely a yummy and delightful treat packed with fiber, vitamins and antioxidants. Indulge in your favorite picks of strawberries, blueberries, and raspberries.

Whole Grains – I love oats in the morning. It's relatively easy to prepare and healthy. A cereal breakfast is packed with fiber that you will end up eating less the entire day, which is great for those who are trying to ward off weight gain.

Fish – It is recommended to eat fish at least twice a week. This is also seen as a healthy option for higher-fat content meats. In addition, this boosts the HDL levels of the physical structure and lower down the triglycerides. This is essentially rich in protein and omega-3 fatty acids that helps tame bad cholesterol levels. Salmon is one healthy choice for this category.

Nuts – Everyone can go crazy over nuts. This is full of antioxidants, which can repair nerve ending and avoid eye damage. This also consequently decreases the risks of cardio vascular diseases as well as trims off excess weight. You can derive great health benefits from seeds, walnuts and nuts that are rich in fiber, magnesium and omega-3 fatty acids.

Dairy Products – I'm a big spender on dairy products. Well, why not? No one is ever too old for milk or yogurt. They're pretty much a good source of vitamin D and calcium that can strengthen the teeth and bones of the body.

Whoa! That is what I call a powerhouse platter. Load your plate with these top 10 superfoods and watch how it gets the reversal done when it comes to lowering your blood glucose and insulin levels to a minimum. I have never thought too that it would be easy to decipher between the "good" food and the "not-so-helpful". The key though is in skillful combination and choosing of food variety that fits above recommendations for diabetic patients.

Having diabetes feels like you're stepping on a ticking bomb. A single mistake can harm your body's systems – and in the process could trigger the bomb inside to explode. Watching every serving you get or the food you eat could be a tedious feat. It troubles me how someone could actually enjoy his food while counting the calories in it.

On the positive note, watching what I eat tells me I am on top of my health. And that is the most important thing for anyone who is suffering such a sensitive condition like diabetes or is pre-diabetic. It's regaining control of the steering wheel – that's the first step to dealing with diabetes. It's not a warzone – not if you think of it. Basically. It's about taking responsibility of your body and making sure you are doing it right this time around.

Sweets That Don't Hurt You

Diabetic patients usually have a thing for sweets. Well, aren't we all? Having diabetes doesn't mean though that you can never take pleasure from a slice of your own birthday cake or have a lollipop every now and then; it simply implies that you have to pick out what sweets to have at appropriate portions. You can easily curb your sweet cravings by going for healthier dessert menus that may seem dangerous (not to mention tempting), but are actually healthy sweets that won't hurt you as much.

Check out these healthy sweet options:

Baked Apples – an apple a day definitely keeps the doctor away. You can slice it into thin wedges and sprinkle it with honey and cinnamon for a health boost. Apples are naturally high in fiber and have very minimal calories. Cinnamon has 'phytochemicals", which radically improves insulin sensitivity, that helps reduce glucose levels.

Berries – one serving of fresh berries usually has a minimum of 60 calories and roughly around 3 grams of protein; plus zero fat. That's a wonderful ratio to have. It's also high in fiber content – a major plus. You can combine blackberries, raspberries, strawberries, and blueberries and soothe your need for sweets without the guilt. Drizzle a teaspoon of honey and you're all set. Honey has only 35 calories per teaspoon so that won't get your sugar levels shoot up that much either.

Dark Chocolates – Who says you can't have coffee? The dark bitter chocolate option has about 170 calories per ounce. Dark chocolate is also proven to help improve blood pressure levels. In fact, study shows that eating 30 grams of dark chocolate daily can help reduce systolic blood sugar pressure. Yet again, the trick here is keeping yourself in line.

See you don't have to completely shut off sweets from your system. That would be weird right? Well, at least from my standpoint as that wouldn't sound healthy too. You can actually substitute and mix sweets and carbohydrates so you get to a certain safety net. However, the trick is to get as natural as possible. Go for fruits and unprocessed ones rather than those that has too many chemical sounding ingredients at their charts.

This means that if you have no choice, it's best to check out the nutrition facts label and just hit straight to the total carbohydrate information to obtain the summary of sugar and starch which can give you the numbers you the numbers you need to decide whether it's a healthy choice or not. Also, servings are very important. You can either combine or swap carbohydrates with sweets as long as meshing up a variety of food groups can give you a much lower sugar and caloric count.

Believe me, I hate numbers too; but if it bears on my health, I would love to do math repeatedly – especially if I get a taste of those delicious dark chocolate and fresh berries. Okay, there you go. Indulge and be tempted. Moreover, don't forget to count.

Chapter 3: Balancing Your Hormones

The Hormone Link

Hormones are chemicals that are used by our body as messengers. Their job is to coordinate each living cell in our body of the many processes they need to have a hand in. These functions range from growth and development to mood swings. That said, they handle a very wide responsibility mainly to keep every tissue and organs in our body working in harmony. Hence, the phrase "I feel like my hormones are out-of-whack" really does hold some bearing.

Most of us do not realize that hormones play a much bigger role in our health. Despite the fact that the society we live in today forces us to become completely out of balance and out of tune, we still fail to develop some habits that would at least lessen the blow of our lifestyle in our health.

As for me, being told that I was pre-diabetic was a wakeup call that I have submerged myself too deep into the hectic lifestyle. Let me look back at what my normal day used to be. I had the regular 9 to 5 job during the weekdays. At work I sit in front of the computer all day to fix the concerns our customers experience with their accounts (I was a bank representative). After work, I'll sit down on my couch and watch sports games or any other TV shows that I've missed through the DVR. Then I spend about 2 hours reading a book until I fall asleep. The next day would look exactly the same.

I'd say the only difference would be how many times I'll be connected to the internet through my smartphone, which I bring with me anywhere. Leisure for me is finding a good spot where there is a strong data signal from my phone network so I could surf the internet on the latest handheld gadget I bought to reassure myself I had a good life.

Being told that I have to deal life with what could be a chronic condition made me step back and look at the bigger picture from atop. From there it's easy to realize that the lifestyle most of us share doesn't fit how our body is organized.

Take a moment and compare your normal day with mine. Even with that short description, do you see so many resemblances?

Let me ask you further:

- Do you have mood swings that often make your personality unpredictable?

- Are you craving for sweets at certain times of the day?

- Do you even get the recommended hours of sleep?

Are you starting to rely too much on substances like coffee, sugar or alcohol just to feel normal?

If so, there's a good chance that your hormones are indeed out of whack.

I asked these questions because these are the same dilemma's I was feeling which I figured are directly linked to the terrible lifestyle I've been keeping for years. From there I learned about hormonal imbalance. And when it comes to diabetes, hormonal imbalance is the main reason for why the condition exists.

Insulin is the hormone we're going to concentrate on. The pancreas secretes it and is responsible in maintaining our body's metabolism in full working condition. Metabolism is a process, which starts from our consumption of food. As we all know, the process of digestion turns the food we eat into chemical compounds so that it could be part of the common building blocks our body uses to restore itself.

Proteins, fats and sugars are the most common life-giving products of digestion. However, there's even a bigger process called metabolism that would include digestion and the actual process of assimilation of these products into the tissues and organs that needs it.

Well, guess what. Insulin is one of the most important gear that will ensure metabolism's clock keeps on ticking. Without it, the entire process takes a detour to nowhere after digestion rather than going into absorption.

When you're trying to battle diabetes, one term you would often hear is Glucose.

What is it? It's the kind of sugar that our body converts the carbohydrates in our food into. Every amount of carbohydrate that we eat gets broken down into glucose. The problem is glucose in large amounts is actually bad for us. It's supposed to be used every time. Our body doesn't like it floating around in our blood because it's toxic.

It should be used as fuel right away or else it would get stored as Glycogen, or in simple terms, fat. Unfortunately, the receptors that converts unused Glucose into fat is easily overwhelmed. Being inactive, uncontrollable consumption of carbs and sugar obviously makes the problem worse.

Here is where it gets even worse. If the pancreas detects that it is unable to suppress the presence of glucose in the bloodstream, it overreacts and releases more insulin. It becomes a viscous cycle when glucose isn't regulated. The body may build up a resistance to insulin. We're now looking at type 2 diabetes - the most common form of this disease.

A healthy body functions as a whole. Hormones are released, as they should at the correct amounts. When one endocrine system (such as the pancreas) becomes imbalance, the entire body suffers. Countless research has linked stress levels as one factor that throws our hormones off balance, which leads to diseases like diabetes.

When you are stressed, cortisol and adrenaline (remember them) are released into the blood stream. They are the hormones ordinarily called upon during situations where actions need to be done on the fly because danger is nearby. Like many of the hormones we've already discussed, if they aren't used up because they normally shouldn't even be there (let's face it, you're not really in physical danger when you get stressed), those hormones end up being more disruptive than helpful.

They actually limit the body's ability to keep our blood sugar in check, raise insulin, limits the thyroids that also reduces our fat burning ability. Being stressed all the time sets off a domino effect that over a long period, always leads to terrible complications.

How do we deal with it? Luckily, I've already been in there and back. In addition, in my journey, I found a good deal of ways on how to effectively overturn the effects of stress in diabetes the natural way. You don't have to turn to drugs to combat stress since we all know its effects. We can all learn from what happened to famous celebrities who became dependent on drugs, which they've apparently started to relieve them of their stress level.

Take Control of Your Carbohydrates Consumption – Diabetes is triggered when our body begins to build up a resistance to insulin. Too much insulin is released as a counterattack to over consumption of sugar, grains and carbohydrates. Therefore, you should restrain yourself from consuming foods with high concentration of these.

Stay Positive – fighting stress by looking at the bright side of things helps lessen tension. It's always nicer if you can keep thoughts that you cherish like family, friends, and places you love close to your heart.

Admit Your Shortcomings – you would be surprised at how something as simple as being nice to yourself can lessen your stress and all the complications that come with it. While I was assessing how I am going to fight diabetes, I noticed that stress mostly came from the pressure I put upon myself. I expected too many results from whatever I was involved in.

Pass On What You Cannot Change Alone – when I was being troubled by diabetes, I noted that much of the stressful situation came from things not really worth my time. You have to learn to distance yourself from the tasks that could lead you feeling stressed even though it really isn't worth the trouble if you think about it. My plan of action in this scenario is to ask myself the following questions:

- Would this be an accomplishment I would like to look back?
- Is there a better way to handle this?
- Now that I have a special burden, is this worth the trouble?

Vent Out To Someone – managing stress doesn't mean you have to bottle it up inside. Don't forget that inside the pressure still builds up. When something is bothering, there's no beating the age-old friend of talking to a real person. I know we're in the internet age and communicating to someone is easy, but have you asked yourself, "when was the last time you really were able to talk to a friend?"

Your friend don't even have to offer any solutions. Simply listening to what you have to say will do. If you're not comfortable with talking to a family member or friend, then there are professionals you could seek for assistance.

Time for Relaxation Becomes 1000x More Important – since being diagnosed as a pre-diabetic, I've used relaxation techniques like yoga, muscle relaxation, and visualization.

Chapter 4: The Role of Sleep in Diabetics

Sleep has gotten a lot of love from the media lately. While it seems elementary, the topic of "what are the consequences of not having enough sleep" is getting a lot of attention simply because everyone feels like they're not getting enough of it.

It's a good thing that science has finally caught up to the rising dilemma of today's world when it comes to our sleeping habits. Time and again, researches have shown how not having enough of affects every aspect of a person's life may it be physical, emotional and mental.

It's on every working person's lips; "I'm not getting the sleep I deserve". What follows are even more clichés that serves as excuse on why we're so desperate such as "I have insomnia, too many distractions; there are kids in the house, etc…

But if we're to go at the bottom of the problem, we'll see that the problem all stems from us cramming too much tasks in the 24 hours that we get in a day.

At the time when I began my battle against diabetes, I was in line to ascend the next higher job position in our company. I was offered a managerial position. The job would have removed me from my desk into a bigger desk, together with a better salary.

If I accept, I wouldn't need to worry about individual customer accounts anymore, instead, the company would expect me to support the performance of 9-12 representatives. I turned the offer down.

Although, the salary was better, it's the only thing tempting with the job offer. Considering the extra condition I recently had to deal with then, the risks outweighs the benefits for me.

When you're struggling with diabetes as well, you should expect that tougher decision would fall your way. And most of the time, you'll have to turn down the ones you would have normally chosen if you were not stricken by diabetes.

Going back to my decision, I knew that the added responsibility as a manager would increase the stress I'm dealing with primarily because it will deprive me more of sleep.

Luckily, I already knew how important sleep was when it's time to make the choice. I knew that I was already in a more important race even more so than my career. And it was a race of reversing the effects of insulin resistance.

Relieving stress and getting enough sleep will boost my chances of winning that race, which I cannot afford to lose.

To get more sleep, you first need to be familiar with the five stages of sleep:

- Stage 1 – this is the stage in our sleep wherein you're not even sure if you're asleep. The term half-asleep may fall under this level. At this stage, the brain starts to weaken its signal that will prompt the rest of the body for its transition to sleep. This period typically lasts only 5-10 minutes.

- Stage 2 – the second stage of sleep lasts around 20 minutes. This is when our body starts to lower down its temperature and heart rate.

- Stage 3 – is what's known to researchers as deep slow sleep. It's at this point when delta waves from the brain starts to seep in. Stage 3 serves as the line between light and deep sleep.

- Stage 4 – this is what's called delta sleep because delta waves (slow brain waves occur). This period lasts approximately 30mins until we get to stage 5.

- Stage 5 – or better known as REM (Rapid Eye Movement) sleep. Although brain activity is at its highest in this point, our body is at its most relaxed state in this stage. Our body restores itself the fastest at this stage and is also when dreams occur. This means that of you haven't dreamt of anything for a long time, you might not have gotten to this point in a while. Level 5 is the last, which means people do not reach this stage through naps. And even with a full night's sleep, this stage only makes up a quarter of that. Therefore, if our sleeping time is shortened, that quarter of a percentage is the first one to get the cut.

I hope that knowing the things above has given you an enhanced sense of appreciation for sleep as I do. I find sleep vital in my fight against diabetes. I wouldn't have won that initial battle if I didn't put enough effort in developing the habits to ensure I get enough sleep.

Here are some tips I've learned along the way to help me doze off.

Have A Consistent Sleeping Pattern – it turns out that our most solid sleep happens when we stay on a schedule. Research approves of this because our body transitions better through the stages of sleep when they occur on consistent hours. We all know that inside we all have our body clock, which appreciates if we don't mess with our sleeping pattern.

Turn the Lights Off Completely – research has also unrivalled that even the slightest light source can interfere with the production of melatonin and serotonin (sleep hormones), which makes us more vulnerable to wake up due to disruptions. Having total darkness by using dark curtains and sleep masks really does have profound effects so that we can reach the deepest stage of sleep.

Avoid High Carbohydrates and Sugars When It's close To Bedtime – doing so raises your blood pressure that makes it harder for the body to release the necessary hormones for sleep.

Keep Your Room Cool – the human body's temperature is at its lowest during deep sleep, which occurs usually during the hours of 10pm – 2am. Making sure that the room is cooler than the body is proven the most conducive temperature for sleep. Research shows that 65 F is the best temperature to reach.

Be Inactive Way before Bedtime – read a book, bathe, do the relaxing activities we've talked about, just don't exercise. You want to do inactive activities before bed because it doesn't impede the production of sleep hormones.

Exercise – during the daytime, when you're not supposed to go to sleep – exercise. Besides the countless benefits that daily exercise brings, it also ensures that the production of sleep hormones is at optimal level.

Avoid Caffeine – you would be surprised at how effective caffeine is able to keep us from dozing. Research has shown that even in small quantities, it is able to inhibit sleep. In fact, even coffee the cup of joe you took at noon may be the reason you're still awake at late nights (depending on your caffeine sensitivity).

Eat a Healthy Diet – staying away from processed foods all day really does help our body at night enter deep sleep stages. As we've said, our eating pattern dictates how successful we are going to be in our fight with diabetes and it shows even on how we can get enough sleep.

Chapter 5: Does Exercise Really Matter?

When it comes to how vital exercise is in fighting diabetes, even the mainstream health care providers recognize how much of an impact exercise can bring. A person who regularly exercises improves his muscle's ability to consume insulin, so over time it helps bring back the state before insulin resistance was even a problem.

Exercise is safe – and is recommended by everyone – from those who pushes for natural medication and even those that go for the synthetic ones. For people with type 2 diabetes, exercise along with diet and stress management can help you take control of your blood sugar levels even if you've already developed complications.

However, if you hold the same lifestyle I was living when I was diagnosed with the dreaded condition, you probably haven't worked in years. If so, don't worry; exercise was a huge obstacle for me too. That's why I needed the assistance of some of my more health inclined friends.

They introduced me to exercises that will make my lifestyle shift a slow transition as I work up. Personally, I kept the thought of doing away with my flab as motivation. You should know that losing excess weight is a commitment you'll going to have to make if you're to walk the same healthier path I chose.

Obesity and diabetes often are linked together. It's often the case of "what came first, the chicken or the egg?" Researches show that not being obese helps mitigate the damage done by diabetes and with constant exercise can actually reverse its effects. Now I'm going to tell you the same exercise tips I was given to help me have the upper hand against diabetes.

Do Quick Workouts – people with diabetes generally have been dormant for the better part of their life. In order to turn things around, they have to become a more active person. Research proves that being an active person means that you at least are working out for 30 minutes every single day. I know how difficult it is to suddenly go 360 on what you've been doing for years, and is in fact the toughest switch I had to make, that's why experts say it's okay to break the 30 minutes into increments that you can handle. If you find it impossible to sustain a half an hour exercise routine in one stretch then try doing quick workouts. As long as it adds up to 30 minutes, it's okay.

Adopt An Overall Active Lifestyle – get a pedometer! It's a device that counts your steps. Having it throughout the day makes you feel motivated because you can gauge in real time the amount of energy you're using versus how much you've consumed. To add to that, research shows that people who use pedometers are able to increase their overall daily activity by 27% on average. That's a whopping figure! When you become a diabetic, far too often people tell us that we need to all of a sudden transform into a different person – a more active person. Simple tricks like prolonging your chores, taking the stairs every time you get the chance, and riding a bike instead of a car to go to places less than 5 miles away helped me a lot in my fight against diabetes and quieting those naggers.

Workout with a Friend – in my case, I would have to say that having 2 friends who works as nurses is one of the largest factors that made me achieve a complete turnaround from my inactive ways. Both of them are living an active lifestyle – they are able to do full marathons, they enjoy biking, hiking and doing anything that would place them outdoors. Their profession has a lot to do with that, but their personality made them choose that profession in the first place I suppose. And I was a lucky beneficiary of their lifestyle. Little by little, the habits of those kind of people will surely trickle down to you. If you can't find friends like that, getting a trainer is an important part of reversing diabetes the natural way.

Set Realistic, Doable Goals – I can't tell you how many diabetics I've met who instead of making progress with exercise and their disease, have regressed because of failed expectations for themselves. Setting specific, attainable goals within the first 3 months is vital. Achieving milestones and the good feeling that comes with breaking personal records are the part of my transformation process I will always look back to as some of the most significant.

Make Your Gadgets Undergo the Same Transformation – when I was still strapped to my desk at work, the apps on my smartphone are for productivity, word processing, and mostly meant for people who plans to sit all day. Now that I've embraced the natural methods of restoring my body, I noticed that my smartphone now is filled with apps used for navigation, training and exercise. The same thing happened to my tablet and laptop. The takeaway of this story is that if you want to undergo an abrupt change in your lifestyle, you'll need all the help you can get – from family, friends and even the tools that you use every day.

Get an Exercise Prescription – not all exercise is the same. They differ in intensity and usefulness. In some cases, an exercise of a certain intensity and when done at a specific time can actually be bad for a diabetic. Your blood sugar can rise during and right after an exercise, which could make the effects of diabetes worse.

Therefore, you need to have your exercise plan approved by a physiologist.

For added motivation, here's a list of benefits a diabetic person could get from exercise:

- The body's use of insulin is maximized
- It helps fight obesity
- It improves muscle strength
- Makes the bones have more density
- Strengthens the heart and lowers blood pressure
- Helps us in avoiding heart diseases by lowering bad cholesterol
- Improves your blood circulation
- Enhances overall metabolism
- Improves brain activity
- Gets rid of anxiety, tension and STRESS

Chapter 6: Natural Ways To Fight Blood Sugar

Reducing Blood Sugar

A person who has diabetes, insulin resistance, or is pre-diabetic like I was, is always thrown into a crash course on how to control our blood sugar. With it, comes the experience of having intense carbs and sugar cravings. Because of the sudden changes we are trying to introduce to our body, the temptation to dip into the old ways is almost unbearable. This is easily one of the lousiest things about being diabetic.

To make matters worse, if a diabetic is to rely on the medications and treatments coming from regular health care providers, it almost always will deplete whatever savings the person possesses. And in most cases, they are veering into unfamiliar and dreadful situations like being stuck in debts.

Research has shown that on average, a person trying to control his blood sugar spends around $6000 annually in order to survive. Conventional health care providers spreads out that figure into monitoring tools, medicines, physician fees, eye exams and other maintenance costs.

Even so, there's something even more frightening. That total doesn't include the amount a diabetic person would most likely spend on treating the complications that often arise from having a type 2 diabetes. Infections due to wounds not healing, poor eyesight, stroke, heart ailments, damage to the liver and kidneys are some of the most common conditions that usually follow diabetes. These complications have led some to believe that the actual cost a diabetic pays his conventional health care provider is double the annual figure we've previously mentioned.

If you're like me who is in a constant brink of becoming diabetic or is already a type 2 diabetic, I'm certain you're well aware of the tug-of-war situation we're engaged in in controlling our blood sugar. After a meal, you check your blood sugar and it's too high so you take in medication. Then after an hour of walking around and exercise, you suddenly feel weird and dizzy then you discover you've overdone it. You've burned too much calories and now you find out you're hypoglycemic. From there you're next move is to consume some carbs or something sweet to compensate the lack energy. That's why it often feels like we're being toyed by our medical bills and our cravings.

I've been struggling with the same dilemma for years. Luckily, I have some more natural remedies to share that are also cheaper alternatives. Just take note that I'm not going to mention the ones that are already set as topics on the previous parts of this book so it doesn't become redundant. Here are unique natural medications that are definitely worth the try (they're cheaper).

Nature do make medication for all sorts of disease – including diabetes. We just need to know which are the ones that are most promising or have already been tried by the most number of people. That process of doing research can be arduous. And so to make your life a bit easier, below is a list of natural supplements that has exceeded my standards:

- Bitter melon
- Magnesium citrate
- Prickly pear cactus
- Bilberry
- Fenugreek
- Ginseng

Drink Coffee – Wait a minute. I know I've already said that drinking coffee can negatively affect a diabetic because it disrupts our sleep pattern. But we cannot ignore the results it has shown in reducing our blood sugar level. The solution? Well, there is decaf coffee available right? Drinking that type doesn't hurt our sleeping pattern, but also allows us to benefit from the anti-oxidants that coffee has a lot it turns out.

Green Tea – drinking tea, particularly green tea reduces a person's blood sugar. Just make sure that it's unsweetened or it would have an adverse effect of course.

Eat Cinnamon – keep a jar of cinnamon in your kitchen to help fight diabetes. It is proven to reduce blood sugar. Sprinkle cinnamon powder to unsweetened food you'll eat. Don't rely on cinnamon rolls though, because the starch on it makes any amount of cinnamon useless.

Drink Red Wine – We've often heard that drinking a glass of wine each day is good for you. It's nice to know that it works for diabetics too. A great explanation I've found is other than red wine being good for our heart; its alcohol content is actually what's delivered the most benefits for diabetic patients.

Someone has explained to me than when our liver has to treat with alcohol, it prioritizes it over its other functions – such as releasing glucose into our blood stream. Hence, you get the idea. Just take caution of drinking too much, as we should also be cognizant of its dangers. A glass a day will suffice. Another thing to keep in mind is the red wine already has some sugar content in it. That means in order for its benefits to take effect, you'll need to skip dessert.

Learn How To Walk It Off – if you're feeling anxiety, it has the same effect as stress. We've already discussed how the feeling of being stressed releases hormones that actually raises a person blood sugar. In cases like this, I find that walking is the best solution. Although it sounds simple, it already incorporates several techniques of how to relieve stress such as breathing at a normal rate instead of the more fluctuating breathing we do when we are feeling anxious.

Chapter 7: Nutrition For Diabetes

Food management is the most important trait to have in diabetes management, aside from regular exercise.

A common belief among diabetes patients (and even to some pre-diabetes) is that when you're diabetic, you have to eat less and consider some foods as off-limits to you. However, this isn't entirely true. In fact, you can still eat all your favorite foods even when you're diabetic. All you need to do is to just watch what you eat, and make substitutions for your favorite recipe if necessary.

Nutrition is still very important, even for diabetics. All it needs is a careful diet plan to ensure the best results.

Protein

Protein helps in the building and repair of muscle tissues in the body. Consumption of protein is necessary, especially for diabetics who exercise, especially heavy ones, protein helps in rejuvenating those damaged muscle parts, and allows growth and expansion of the muscles in the body.

Most sources of protein, especially meats, also have a good amount of fat in them. Therefore, regulation of the consumption of these foods is very important, to reduce the intake of fat in your body. If you decide on going for the meat route, always choose the "lean" cuts of either pork or beef, like pork loin or sirloin.

These types of meat cuts give the most amount of protein, while still having the least amount of fat out of any other variety. If you want to consume poultry meats, like chicken or turkey, make sure to always remove the skin from them, since the skin part is where most amounts of fats lie.

Fish and some vegetable are the recommended sources of protein for most, since most of them, especially those of the tuna or salmon variety, also contain omega-3, the so-called "good fats", which actually helps in keeping the heart healthy and reducing the risks of stroke, heart attack and diseases in which diabetics are likely prone to.

Milk and other daily products are also good sources of protein as well as other vitamins and minerals. However, non-fat or low-fat milk is very much recommended to reduce fat intake.

For serving sizes, the recommended sizes for any kind of meat is around 3 ounces per serving, or the size of the deck of cards. For fish, two to three times a week is the recommended serving.

Carbohydrates, or what I keep mentioning as "carbs", are the main nutrient that diabetics should closely monitor. Carbohydrates turn to blood glucose or fat when consumed. Having too much of these carbs raises the risk of diabetes and obesity. However, having too little of these might lessen your overall energy.

The key here is determining the type of carbs that you need to consume. Whole grain foods are better than processed ones because they contain "complex" carbohydrates. These types of carbohydrates take longer for the body to break down; regulating your blood sugar levels and helping your body feel satisfied and filled.

Good sources of healthy carbohydrates include root crops like potatoes, whole grain products, beans, and oats. Whole grain and oats are essentially very important because not only do they contain carbohydrates, but they also contain dietary fiber, a very important nutrient that contributes to digestive health while keeping your intestines clean from toxin buildup.

Vitamins & Minerals

There are different kinds of vitamins and minerals around today, and all of them play an important role in the health of the body. From vitamin A that helps in improving eyesight, to Zinc, every one of them needs to be taken by the body.

Unfortunately, most people fail to meet the recommended nutrient levels for these kinds of vitamins and minerals. This is because not all of the vitamins and minerals are found in the food that we commonly eat. Therefore, a balanced diet and careful meal planning are very essential to make sure you get everything you need.

Vitamins and minerals are commonly found in different foods around, but the richest sources come from different vegetables and fruits, especially from leafy vegetables, different citrus fruits, and berries. Whole grains are also excellent sources of vitamins because they contain the germ and the bran, which houses different nutrients. Furthermore, vegetable and fruits are also rich in fiber for the body, and berries contain a very important nutrient for all of us: antioxidants.

Fats

Contrary to popular belief, not all fats are unhealthy. Fats that come from meat products, like beef, chicken, and pork, are unhealthy, and contribute to the risk of heart problems, which are common among diabetics. To avoid this, always choose leaner cuts of pork, beef, or lamb, and always remove the skin of chicken before cooking them.

Healthy fats, on the other hand, are commonly found in fish, nuts, as well as different plant oils. These actually reduces the risk of heart problems, by keeping the blood vessels healthy and free from bad fat buildup. It's important to consider adding these fats to your daily diet, even in small amounts. Olive oil or vegetable oil is the perfect substitute for recipes that need some oil, so consider stocking up on these kinds of oils instead.

The Perfect Meal Plan for Diabetics

A perfect meal for diabetics, like any other meal plan, should provide all the above nutrients in one serving. Careful planning is thus essential when preparing your food to make sure that you're getting all the nutrients you need.

Food handling and preparation are also important, as mishandling of food can cause them to lose some of their nutrients. In general, choose only the freshest kinds of food available on the market, and proper cooking methods must be followed to ensure that the nutrients I the food stay intact.

Of course, care must also be followed to make sure that you're only eating the right portions of food, so that you don't run the risk of obesity. Therefore, before starting out your own diet plan, it's very important to first consult your local doctor or nutritionist whenever possible, so that they may give you the proper guidelines in starting your meal plan.

Chapter 8: Monitoring Your Blood Sugar Levels

Blood sugar monitoring is very important for diabetes and pre-diabetes patients, especially if you take constant medication to be able to control your blood sugar.

While medication helps in regulating your blood levels, and thus control the symptoms of diabetes, there's always a chance that your blood sugar may become too low than the recommended one. This condition is known as hypoglycemia (as opposed to hyperglycemia, the abnormal rise of blood sugar levels, from which diabetes occurs), and can also cause some complications to the diabetes patient, like sudden weakness and even impairment of several bodily functions.

Therefore, a regularly scheduled blood sugar test is equally important as the medication itself.

Glucose Test

For those who are showing symptoms of diabetes, but still aren't sure if they have indeed the disease, taking a glucose test is the first step for detection. A glucose test is a process to determine the amount of blood glucose (blood sugar) levels, thus, one can have a general idea if they already have diabetes, or showing signs of it. It generally involves having the patient submit a sample of their blood to a doctor, which is then taken to their medical laboratory for further testing.

There are several different types of glucose tests, and while the general process is the same, the reference values for each differ. The general rule of thumb is, for more accurate results, doctors will do two or more of these tests to patients.

(Values come from the guidelines references by the American Diabetes Association).

Fasting Blood Sugar (FBS), or Fasting Plasma Glucose (FPG) – This glucose test is used to determine the blood sugar level of individuals during a state of fast, that is, they haven't consumed anything. Before the test is conducted, the patient is instructed to go fasting for 8 to

12 hours. During that fasting period, the patient must not consume anything at all, from any kind of food, even water. Breaking the fast during this period may show inaccurate results for the test.

Since this glucose test assumes that the patient hasn't consumed anything for an extended period, reference levels for this are lower than other type of tests.

Normal Levels: 4 to 7 mmol/l (milimoles per liter) or 72 to 126 mg/dl (milligrams per decilitre), 3.9 to under 5.5 mmol/l (milimoles per liter) or 70.2 to 100 mg/dl (milligrams per deciliter) after a 12-hour fast.

Diabetes Risk (these needs constant monitoring): 5.5 to 7 mmol/l 101-125mg/dl) and above.

Postprandial Glucose Test – this glucose test is administered to patients to determine their blood sugar levels after a meal.

A healthy person's blood sugar level rises slightly after eating a meal. After two hours, blood sugar level returns to normal levels.

Postprandial glucose tests are done to patients two hours after they have eaten a full meal. For reference, post prandial glucose levels under 180 mg/dl and preprandial plasma glucose between 90-130 mg/dl are considered healthy and normal. Any other values higher than that, and the patient is at risk of diabetes.

Glucose Tolerance Test – In this test, the doctors instruct the patients to ingest a certain dosage of glucose (primarily in liquid form) and blood samples are then taken two hours later for testing.

This test is quite similar to the previous tests for diabetes, except it also tests the patient for insulin resistance, and even reactive hypoglycemia. Thus, this is usually administered to patients to check for type 1 diabetes.

To prepare for the test, it's recommended for patients to not resist intake of any food that are rich in carbohydrates for days, or even weeks, before the test is done. 8 to 12 hours before the test, the patient is then required o fast (though water is allowed).

This test has many different variations over the years, ranging from the glucose dosage intake, to different administrations. Sometimes, this test is now expanded to check for many other substances other than blood sugar levels.

Random Glucose Test – the glucose test is administered to a patient at any time necessary, most commonly after a recent meal. Because of this, the reference values for this are much higher than the other tests, with 80 to 140 mg/dl (3.9 – 7.8 mmol/l) being considered as normal, between 140 – 200 mg/dl is considered pre-diabetes, and 2200 mg/dl and higher is considered diabetic.

This type of test produces the least accurate results, however, patients are still recommended to take other tests in addition to this.

Glucose Testing at Home

You can also administer testing your blood sugar levels. This is done through the usage of an instrument called a "glucose meter". This is very important, especially if you need to monitor your blood sugar levels regularly, due to several factors, as well as for the patient to understand the effects of diet and exercise on blood sugar management.

The reference levels used for the tests involving the glucose meter are almost the same as the tests done in the hospital, with several factors influencing the target range. These include age, diabetes severity, complications, disease duration, etc…

The frequency in which you have to test your blood sugar levels depends on the type of diabetes that you have.

For Type 1 Diabetes Patients: Doctors will usually advice patients to monitor their blood sugar levels at least three or more times a day, usually before and after a meal, before and after an exercise routine, and before bedtime. Monitoring is also essential if you are ill, or if you're going to change your routine as well as medication.

For Type 2 Diabetes Patients: Depending on the insulin dosage that the patients take, doctors usually advice patients to monitor their blood sugar levels once or several times daily; often before meals, or after an 8 hour fast. However, if the patient is managing their diabetes condition with non-insulin medications or with only diet and exercise, then the patient doesn't need to monitor it daily.

In order to achieve accurate results with the glucose meter, proper handling and maintenance is advised.

Follow the instructions set by the user manual of the device for proper usage of the meter. Make sure to always wash your hands with soap and water before usage.

Not all test strips are compatible with your glucose meter. Only buy test strips that are compatible with yours.

Run quality checks on your glucose meter regularly. Also, don't forget to clean them.

Always consult the use manual for further troubleshooting instructions.

Test strips should be stored as directed by the manual. Used strips should be disposed of immediately. Do NOT use expired test strips.

Always bring your glucose meter during your trips to the doctor, so that he may address any questions and to properly demonstrate the use of the meter.

Epilogue

This book is written with the joy of having confirmed that switching over to the more natural ways of fighting diabetes is more enjoyable. I wrote this book with the hope that it would serve as a contagious reason why no-one who is facing the same dilemma I have with diabetes, should give up a significant part of their normal lives in battling the disease.

Inside, there are ample lessons to be learned about how to trim down the factors that would cause the disease to get worse. Also, there are as many tips on how to naturally reverse the effects of diabetes.

We've crossed the major factors that one should mould in your favour like sleep, activities, and eating habits. Together, they form the major chunk of a person's lifestyle that needs to be tweaked to lower a diabetes patient's reliance with traditional medication that occurs from conventional health care providers.

The lessons you have learned will lower down your maintenance cost; will let you take control of your medication and ultimately improve the quality of your life.

I also ensured to not only pour out instructions to you, but to also include the physiological information of every tip. That way, you'll also recognize the reasoning on why you should not skip that certain step. Another benefit of knowing the insides of every point is so that you can easily teach it to your loved one who might also be suffering the same condition.

I know that sticking with everything that I've indicated in this book is not easy. Especially when the world we're living in doesn't apply the same rigid standards I'm asking you to embrace.

Serving a certain dish that's good for you instead of what everyone else in the room expects is close to impossible since I'm asking you to do this everyday. That's why I've written this is the sequence of how I applied it in my life as well. This a gradual journey. One that I hope you'd grow more comfortable in, as I did.

We Want Your Feedback on This Book!

Our main purpose is to make sure that our readers get value from the books we publish and that they have a good experience with all of our products. We are always working to improve our books and other products with every revision and update.

Every piece of feedback makes a difference in this process. And we would appreciate yours as well - whether it is good or bad.

Please take one minute to let us know what you thought by following this link:

http://checkmatemg.com/feedbackdiabetes/